Keto Diet:

Delicious Recipes To Lose Weight, Boost Your Metabolism, And Cleanse Your Body From The Inside Out

Sarah Wilson

presented is without assurance regarding its continued validity or interim quality. Trademarks that mentioned are done without written consent and can in no way be considered an endorsement from the trademark holder.

Table of Contents

Introduction

I want to thank you and congratulate you for downloading this book.

This book contains proven steps and strategies on how to carry out a ketogenic diet without starving yourself in the process.

The prospect of dieting may seem to be daunting. With so many horror stories about the experience, some people understandably want to avoid it at all costs. Perhaps, even you have tried it but opted to stop due to the headaches, hunger, and discomfort you felt during the cleansing period.

But because you are reading this, there's probably a tiny voice in

your head that says you should think about trying it again – that

perhaps, there really is something to dieting!

In this book, you will get new and helpful insights about the practice. This does not intend to belie what others experienced. This focuses more on why you should diet, how you should do it correctly, and how to use the principles of the keto diet to do it.

There are a plethora of cleansing products, services and programs out there, but this book mainly explores a 15-day ketogenic dieting program. Ketogenic diet, simply known as keto diet, is getting more popular in recent years. You will find out how beneficial it is as a diet and as a cleansing program with the help of this book.

This book also addresses the top problem that many people

associate with dieting: the limited number of meals you can devour on your cleansing period. Herein, you can find over a hundred recipes with meat, seafood and vegetable as the main ingredients. There are also numerous ideas for your snack time.

With the information you can gain from this book, your cleansing period does not have to be a daunting experience. If you strictly follow the 15-day dieting program, it will surely be a nourishing and relieving experience.

Thanks again for downloading this book. I hope you enjoy it!

Chapter 1: Why Keto

"It is just another fad diet." This might be your first thought about the keto diet – and you're not alone. It's just hard to get into a diet that claims that eating a high fat diet fat will help you lose excess weight.

Even Hollywood celebrities rave about how they shaved off some pounds by going keto, but celebrities are not exactly the ideal role models when it comes to fitness. Their bankability depends on their looks so they invest a lot in fitness. they often have an image to maintain. However, they might have gotten it correct this time as the diet they are talking about is actually backed by science.

The keto diet, more formally known as ketogenic diet, is low in carbohydrates, moderate in proteins and high in fats. It is often likened to other popular diets such as the Atkins diet and the Low-Carbohydrate, High-Fat (LCHF) diet. But unlike the two, keto does not suggest boosting protein intake to make up for the reduced amount of carbohydrates on the diet.

The Importance of a Low-Carbohydrate Diet

Carbohydrates, proteins and fats are the three major nutrients needed by the body in great amounts for energy, growth, repair and sustenance. Also called the three macronutrients, they make up the majority of a diet. Minerals and vitamins are the micronutrients required by the body but only in trace amounts.

Fruits, breads, cereals, pastas, soft drinks, and other

carbohydrate-rich foods make up the typical modern diet. During digestion, carbohydrates are turned into their simplified form, glucose (also known as blood sugar). A typical diet composed of the aforementioned foods prompts the body to utilize glucose as its main fuel.

Now, many people mistakenly think that because carbohydrate is a macronutrient, it should be okay to consume plenty of it. The truth is that, for the most part, ingesting too much carbs isn't good for you. Most of the carbohydrates we consume in food are sugars (a very small amount covers fiber). As you know, too much sugar in your body increases your risk to heart and kidney diseases. You become more vulnerable to hypertension and stroke as well.

Fatigue, headaches, problematic vision, and intensified thirst are some of the symptoms of hyperglycemia, or the condition of having high blood sugar level. Instead of just managing the signs, you should treat the main cause of the problem. The good news is that hyperglycemia can be reversed and avoided. If the diet triggered the excess sugar levels in your bloodstream, you can also find the solution in your diet.

How the Keto Diet Works

The keto diet supports the idea of reducing carbohydrate intake which leads to the decrease of glucose in the body. As the amount of glucose goes down, the body has to look for another source of fuel to function. This is where the increase in fat intake becomes valuable.

Proteins are mainly for growth, repair and maintenance while fats are typically stored if there is too much carbohydrates in the diet. In keto diet, the body makes use of the stored fats as source of fuel. The liver gathers fatty acids from body fats and breaks them down into ketones.

When ketones successfully replace glucose as the primary source of fuel for the brain and cells alike, the body is deemed to be in a state of ketosis. Ketogenic diet got its name after its aim: to put the body in the state of ketosis.

If you decide to commit to the diet, you will need ketone test strips to find out whether or not your body has achieved ketosis. You can adjust your fat and carbohydrate intake based on the results of your tests. The test strips are based on the ketone content in your blood or urine.

For beginners, the ideal ratio between fat intake and the combined protein and carbohydrate intake is 2:1. Some practitioners go as far as 4:1. The extra proteins in your diet can be converted into glucose so you should still keep your protein intake in moderate amounts.

What Keto Diet Is Not

Aside from the studies that prove its efficiency, healthcare professionals and fitness experts recommend keto diet because it does not require you to completely remove a specific macronutrient from your diet, such as in the case of no-fat diets. It does not require you to totally eliminate carbohydrate as well. You can still eat carbohydrates (and you should) but only at low amounts.

Just because fruits are healthy does not mean that all of them are okay to eat when you're in a keto diet. A glass of 100% fruit juice is not recommended in the diet due to its high carbohydrate content. However, adding a teaspoon of lemon juice in your keto meal is not likely to be as bad as downing an entire glass of juice drink. In this sense, the diet is less restrictive but still beneficial.

Finally, if you're trying to engage in heavy physical training, this diet regimen is not for you. Carbohydrates are still the body's main energy source and going on a strict keto diet will not allow you to have sufficient carb intake.

Benefits of the Keto Diet

Lowering your carbohydrate intake and putting your body in a state of ketosis with the help of the keto diet lead to numerous health benefits. The most prominent of which is efficient weight loss.

Under ketosis, your body basically burns stored fat for fuel. As a result, you lose the weight that comes with those fats. A low blood sugar level also means a decrease in the production of insulin, the hormone responsible for fat storage. This helps you maintain your weight. Weight loss and low blood sugar levels result to other advantages such as the reduced risk of developing diabetes, cancers and cardiovascular diseases.

Additionally, ketones are proven by studies to be better than glucose when it comes to your mental health. With ketones, you will crave less for food which keeps distractions at bay and prevents you from getting easily irritable. You will experience fewer and less severe migraine attacks as well.

The keto diet is also advantageous in the management of epilepsy, acne and polycystic ovarian syndrome (PCOS). In fact, it has been the recommended diet for individuals with epilepsy for several decades. This only proves that the diet is not another fad diet that celebrities are simply popularizing in the past few years.

Challenges You'll Have to Face

There will always be a set of challenges that you have to deal with when you decide to shift to a new diet. In keto, the main drawback is that you have to say goodbye to your everyday meals full of pastas, sweets and flavored drinks. However, you can comfort yourself with the plethora of delicious keto meals you can make at home.

During the first few weeks of dieting, you might experience some side effects as well. Some got the so-called keto flu and complained about their lower energy levels.

These should not discourage you from adhering to the diet as these effects are temporary. Furthermore, you have to understand that your body is in an adjustment phase. You have to press on if you want to reap the benefits of the diet.

Chapter 2: Why Cleanse

Over time, your body accumulates toxins from the air you breathe, the water you drink, the food you eat, the products you use and the thoughts you entertain. The human body is designed in such a way that it can filter and expel toxins by exhaling, perspiring, urinating and defecating. However, it still needs some help to keep the organs responsible for excretion in their optimal condition.

In this book, the focus is on the foods and drinks you consume. Regardless of your diet, your body gathers some toxins which are often stored in the intestinal tract. This does not mean that adhering to a diet is useless. This simply entails that you have to prevent the possible accumulation of too much toxins in your digestive system. When it comes to this task, cleansing can be helpful.

What Cleansing is All About

In general, cleansing is the act of removing the toxins, waste and harmful microorganisms out of the body. There are different cleansing methods and products you can try. There is yoga for toxic thoughts. There are exfoliating creams for your dead skin cells. There are also cleansing juices intended for your intestinal tract.

The term detoxification, or simply detox, is often used interchangeably with cleansing. While both aims to expel toxins, the latter tends to be more inclusive as it covers the removal of non-beneficial bacteria and parasites.

Cleansing is a great help in preventing health conditions such as allergies, dementia, constipation, frequent inflammations, heavy metal poisoning and colon cancer. It improves your energy, focus and mood as well. Most importantly, it improves your metabolism and keeps your intestines healthy, resulting to the quick and efficient absorption of nutrients needed by the other organs in the body.

Sources of Toxins and Parasites in the Intestinal Tract

Many of the products you can buy in a grocery store are prepared, processed and packed using chemicals. When ingested, these chemicals become the number one source of toxins in your intestines.

If the produce you bought is cultivated using non-organic farming methods, the toxins you may get will be much more than the ones you can get from organic produce.

As your intestinal tract is burdened by more toxins, it becomes a more conducive habitat to harmful microorganisms. Regular bowel movement helps keep this problem at bay. However, it is not enough to avoid the negative effects of accumulating toxins and parasites. If you suffer from frequent constipation, inflammation and infections despite following a healthy diet like keto, your body might be telling you to pause for a moment and let your digestive system recover.

Cleansing Products versus Cleansing Diets

Just like in anything else, marketers took notice of the increasing interest in cleansing. As a result, they invented products that target those who want to cleanse their bodies in a more convenient manner. You might have heard of juice cleanse before. There are over-the-counter drugs for deworming as well.

There is no doubt that opting for cleansing products is highly convenient. In the case of deworming, products are even more effective than diets. However, using cleansing products should be accompanied by a diet. Furthermore, these products should only be used a few times while you are under a cleansing program.

A cleansing program is composed of meal plans for a certain period of time. Everyone should cleanse twice or thrice a year. The duration of cleansing differs from one program to another. The main factor often considered in the duration is the type of toxic waste or parasites a program aims to remove. Some are as short as three days while others go for as long as a month. In the succeeding chapter, you will learn how to carry out a 15-day cleansing program.

Why Keto Cleanse

Cleansing is like resetting your intestinal tract. It is a good way to introduce your body in a new diet. In the previous chapter, you learned the benefits of following a keto diet. If you want to try it (or give it another try in case you tried it before but stopped), cleansing will help you adjust to the diet. The cleansing program for you should be based on the principle of the keto diet.

Aside from helping you adjust to the diet, a keto cleansing program speeds up your weight loss. It lessens the burden on your liver as well. The liver is another organ responsible in the management of toxins in the body. It may take you a longer time to achieve a state of ketosis due to the amount of detoxifying work that your liver has to do. With a keto cleansing program, your liver can focus on the conversion of fatty acids into ketones instead of working too much on toxic waste.

Unlike other cleansing programs, keto emphasizes the consumption of solid foods, not just water, juices or soups in its entire duration. You are not going to starve yourself. In this book, you will find plenty of keto recipes to help you get by each day in your cleansing period.

Chapter 3: The 15-Day Keto Cleansing Program

The 15-day keto cleansing program combines the basic principles behind the keto diet and cleansing: the consumption of low-carbohydrate, moderate-protein and high-fat meals made from plants grown organically, animals fed only with grass and/or grains, as well as fish and seafood caught in the wild.

This cleansing program stands out from the rest because it does not highlight the use of fruits and fruit juices which are known to have high carbohydrate content.

A 15-day cleansing program is more manageable than others that require 30 days. The former forces your body to adjust to the cleansing diet and go back to your regular diet more quickly. Despite the shorter duration, you can gain the same benefits that a 30-day program offers so long as you stick to the meal plans.

Day 1-7

Enjoy the first week of the cleansing program by switching between high-fat meat and seafood dishes with a serving of vegetables for your lunch and dinner. Start each day with a keto drink and/or soup. You can make your own keto sauces for your dishes and snacks alike. If you are going to eat fruit, you should opt for avocados because it is rich in fats and low in carbohydrates. You may consume strawberries, blackberries and raspberries as snacks but only in fewer amounts.

Day 8-15

For the second week, you have to double your keto drink and soup intake as cleansing requires liquids to speed up the flushing of toxins out of your body. Instead of meat, fish and seafood, your lunches and dinners should feature vegetable dishes. You can eat up to three handfuls of macadamia, pecan or Brazil nuts a day for your snacks. When choosing your snacks for the eight to fifteenth days, always go for something with fewer ingredients.

Your initial hunt for the ingredients is going to be a stressful task because you cannot just buy any meat or produce. You will find a more detailed guideline about the foods you can take and the foods you should avoid in the next chapter. Shopping tips are included therein as well.

Who Should Not Follow this Cleansing Program?

The keto diet, along with the cleansing program, is not for everyone though. If you are a breastfeeding mother, you have to wait until your child can depend on solid food for nutrients instead of breast milk. A low-carbohydrate and moderate-protein diet can affect your milk production so it is best to avoid it first.

Also, you are not supposed to follow the diet and the cleansing program if you are currently on medications for hypertension or for type II diabetes. Consult your primary care provider about your hypertension or diabetes management and the possibility of adhering to keto diet if you want to try it.

Managing the Possible Side Effects

During the 15-day keto cleansing program, you might experience a sudden drop in your performance. If you are working out, try to reduce the intensity or volume of your training.

Energy drinks are going to be tempting but never rely on them because of their carbohydrate content and artificial flavoring. Your cleansing attempt will turn out to be futile if you get more toxins from the said drink.

You may eat a bit more of low-carbohydrate foods in case the first few days become too grueling. Aside from that, you should make sure that you get enough rest so you will not feel easily tired during the cleansing period.

Additional Tips

You do not need to wait for your cleansing period to start preventing the accumulation of toxins in your body. Days before you commit to cleansing, make sure to reduce your caffeine and sugar intake. Aside from lessening the toxins that your body will gain, this helps minimize the severity of headaches on the first few days of cleansing.

During your cleansing period, avoid dining out as much as possible. Spend the time preparing your own meals instead. By doing so, you know the ingredients that form part of the foods you eat. You can assure the cleanliness of your meal preparation as well.

It pays to minimize your social engagements, too. This gives you fewer reasons to spend time on restaurants and bars. Anyway, the cleansing period only lasts for 15 days so you are not likely to miss out on a lot of events.

When setting the dates for your cleansing period, take note of the commitments, events, and holidays that may coincide in those days. It is best to kick off cleansing on a Thursday or Friday. If you have slow metabolism, your body may not react to the diet change right away. You may feel the effects though starting on the second to fourth day. Those days are going to be tough so it is good idea to be at home during those days.

Finally, prepare a week-long meal plan instead of deciding your meals right before you cook them. You can save some bucks if you just buy what you need for your week-long menu. Additionally, you can opt to make two or more servings of one dish and save the leftovers for the next day. This makes your meal preparation less time-consuming than necessary.

Chapter 4: Preparing Your Kitchen For Keto Cleansing

Sometimes, a new diet requires a pantry overhaul. If yours is filled with too much junk foods and processed goods, you have to toss them out to get rid of the temptation. Give them away or consume them before you undergo the 15-day cleansing period. As you eliminate the unhealthy foods in your kitchen, you need to fill your pantry and fridge with high-fat and low-carbohydrate foods.

High-Fat Group

Dietary fats are not as evil as what you might have conceived before. As a macronutrient, they have important functions in the body; among their functions is the absorption of some vitamins and minerals. As your body loses stored fats during ketosis, dietary fats can help replace the lost fats and sustain your state of ketosis.

High-fat foods from animal sources include ghee, grass-fed butter, grass-fed cheese, grass-fed beef, grass-fed offal, free-range pork, free-range chicken and free-range eggs. Wild herring, mackerel, trout and salmon are rich in the said macronutrient as well. For the plant-based high-fat ingredients and snacks, you can choose from avocados, olive oil, macadamia nuts, flaxseeds and sunflower seeds—all of which should be organic.

Low-Carbohydrate Group

Your body still needs carbohydrates to transform fats into ketones. Therefore, you should not ditch the macronutrient entirely but do not consume much of it as well.

Many of the aforementioned high-fat foods are known to be low in carbohydrates. Other low-carbohydrate foods include: raspberries, strawberries, blackberries, celery, lettuce, cucumber, pepper, spinach, asparagus, kale, chives, Bok Choy, endive, chard, bamboo shoots, and radicchio. Prawns belong to this group as well.

Moderate-Protein Group

As for your protein needs, you can simply satisfy it with eggs. These are one of the richest sources of the macronutrient. Gelatin can be a source of both proteins and fats. If you are working out, this food group helps you sustain your muscle mass during your cleansing period.

Spices and Condiments

Most herbs and spices are well-suited to the keto cleansing program. Although fruit juices are not recommended as your beverage, you can have lemon or lime juice as part of the ingredients for a dish.

Instead of ready-made condiments, you may also opt to make your own. You can make your own mayonnaise for example. You can replace traditional breading with ground pork rinds as well. Say goodbye to refined sugar and brown sugar. Go for low-carb sweeteners like Erythritol, Swerve and Stevia instead. With these condiments, you can be sure to have a diet that is efficient in cleansing yet flavorful.

Beverages

Liquids are as important as the solid foods you consume to flush out the toxins out of your body. Not all beverages are good during the cleansing period though. As always, water is still the best drink out there. Aside from being the purest among all beverages, it is also the cheapest yet remains the most efficient. If you want, you can make infused water for a more satisfying way of drinking. Certain kinds of teas are also worth ingesting during your cleansing period because of their antioxidants. You can make smoothies for more delicious drinks.

Foods to Avoid

Without a doubt, the number one food group that you have to avoid when under a keto diet or cleanse is any food rich in carbohydrates. Among them are grains and their derivatives. No rice, corn, cereals, pastas, breads and biscuits as your body undergoes cleansing.

Well-loved tropical fruits like banana, papaya, mango and pineapple also have high carbohydrate content which makes them not ideal for a keto cleanse. Snacks, beverages and other food products made out of high-carbohydrate fruits should not also form part of your meals during the cleansing period. Other high-carbohydrate foods you should avoid include: potatoes, sweet potatoes, yams, parsnips, carrots, soy and soy products, and soft drinks.

Products of non-organic farming methods must be avoided as well. Apart from plant produce, these also include pork, chicken and fish from farms. Many of today's farms feed synthetic foods to the said animals. Such leave toxins in the body of the pigs, chicken and fishes which they carry even after being slaughtered or caught.

Furthermore, you should not use margarine and any other product made with preservatives, flavorings, food coloring and artificial sweeteners. Regarding the beverages, alcohol must be avoided during the cleansing period.

Shopping Tips

Before you shop for the ingredients, decide what to prioritize: will it be the recipe or the availability? In the next chapter, you can browse among different recipes. If you focus on availability, you can save money, time and effort when shopping. The challenge herein is to find the right recipe that suits most of the foods on season. After making a list of foods that are on season, take notes of the meals you can prepare using them. List down the additional ingredients you will need as well.

In contrast, focusing on recipes makes it easy to set the schedule for each meal. The downside is the cost of some off-season goods. When you can hardly decide between the two, weigh on the foods you are looking forward to eat which can be included in a keto cleanse diet. Are they mostly on-season foods or not? Finalize your cleansing meal plan afterwards.

Once you decided where to focus, download a shopping list template or make your own. It should have columns dedicated for meat, fish, sea food, vegetables, fruits, dairy, condiments, spices, beverages, baking goods and other essentials that do not fall under any of the aforementioned categories.

As much as possible, go for locally and organically grown produce. Visit a nearby farmer's market to shop for fruits, vegetables, meat, offal, eggs, herbs and spices. When it comes to meat, you can try different cuts if you want to buy something more economical. Fatty and bony cuts for examples are cheaper than other popular cuts.

Go to your preferred grocery store for the other products not available on the farmer's market. If there are no grass-fed meat, offal, butter and ghee, you can opt for their pasture-raised counterparts. Pasture-raised products are less expensive. However, the cows where they come from are fed with other foods apart from grasses. Nevertheless, this should not cause any alarm because during winter months, grasses or hay supply are quite limited so the cows are fed with other foods.

When you shop, whether on the local farmer's market or grocery store, always bring a copy of your shopping list and stick to the items you are supposed to buy. Avoid lingering for too long in each aisle in the grocery store to prevent being tempted by carbohydrate-rich products. Read the labels carefully as well. You may also buy in bulk especially for items like eggs and olive oil, but be mindful of their expiration dates.

Additionally, you should avoid pre-packaged meals. Different kinds of salads are available in many grocery stores today. Pre-packaged keto meals are also available on the market today but only in a few areas. They are certainly a convenient option if you have limited cooking skills. However, you will have no idea about some of the ingredients used in their preparation.

Food Preparation Tools

Just to be clear, you do not need to buy a lot of tools before you start cleansing. However, when you decide to commit to a healthy way of eating, you might want to invest in the following kitchen equipment: pressure cooker, slow cooker, dehydrator, immersion blender and food processor.

For now, make sure you have the following tools in your kitchen: skillets, saucepans, pots, cookie sheets, baking sheets, parchment paper, foil, bowls, jars, containers, wooden spoons, silicone spatulas, tongs, strainers, measuring spoons and cups, digital kitchen scales, cutting boards, knives and a dedicated sharpener, graters, and kitchen shears.

It also pays to have a steamer basket and spiralizer (also called spiral slicer) for your fruit or vegetable preparation. Additionally, you should invest on lunch boxes that you can proudly and gladly bring in your office so you can avoid dining out or opting for fast-food.

Chapter 5: Keto Cleanse Recipes

Keto Cleanse Drinks

Strawberry Cream Smoothie

Prep Time: 5 minutes

Serving Size: 40g; **Serves:** 1

Ingredients:

5 strawberries

3 tablespoons heavy cream

1 teaspoon low-carb sweetener (Erythritol, Swerve or Stevia)

Directions:

1. Blend the strawberries, heavy cream, and sweetener until smooth.

Raspberry Cheese Smoothie

Prep Time: 5 minutes

Serving Size: 40g; **Serves:** 2

Ingredients:

½ cup raspberries

1 cup almond milk

1 fluid ounce cream cheese

1 teaspoon low-carb sweetener (Erythritol, Swerve or Stevia)

Directions:

1. Blend the raspberries, almond milk, cream cheese and sweetener until smooth.

Strawberry Lemonade

Prep Time: 10 minutes

Serving Size: 40g; **Serves:** 6

Ingredients:

1 pint strawberries, sliced

6 lemons, juiced

8 cups water

2 cups ice cubes

½ teaspoon Stevia

Directions:

1. Mix the lemon juice, water, ice cubes and Stevia in a large pitcher.

2. Add the strawberry slices and stir. Allow the flavor to sit for 15 minutes.

Berry Spinach Smoothie

Prep Time: 10 minutes

Serving Size: 40g; **Serves:** 2

Ingredients:

2 cups mixed berries (preferably blackberries, strawberries and raspberries)

2 cups spinach

1 cup water

½ cup crushed ice (optional)

Directions:

1. Put the first three ingredients in a blender. Add crushed ice if you prefer a cold smoothie.

2. Blend until smooth.

Nutty Spinach Smoothie

Prep Time: 5-10 minutes

Serving Size: 40g; **Serves:** 2

Ingredients:

10 almonds (preferably pre-chopped)

2 Brazil nuts (preferably pre-chopped)

2 cups spinach

1 cup unsweetened coconut milk

Directions:

1. If you have no pre-chopped almonds and Brazil nuts, you can opt for the whole nuts and crush them on your own. You may use a rolling pin and a cutting board to do so. You may also use a food processor.

2. Once you have the crushed nuts, put them in the blender along with the spinach and coconut milk.

3. Blend until smooth.

Tangy Green Smoothie

Prep Time: 15 minutes

Serving Size: 40g; **Serves:** 4

Ingredients:

4 cups kale

1 avocado, peeled, halved and pitted

½ cucumber

1½ cups water

2 tablespoons lemon juice

Directions:

1. Blend the avocado, cucumber and lemon juice first.

2. Once pureed, add the kale and water.

3. Blend until smooth.

Cold and Citrusy Cucumber Celery Smoothie

Prep Time: 10 minutes

Serving Size: 40g; **Serves:** 2

Ingredients:

2 celery heart stalks, chopped

½ cucumber, peeled, chopped and seeded

1 tablespoon lime juice

¼ cup water

¼ cup crushed ice

Directions:

1. Blend all the ingredients until smooth.

2. Strain to make it a juice.

Mint Green Smoothie

Prep Time: 15 minutes

Serving Size: 40g; **Serves:** 2-3

Ingredients:

6 mint leaves

3 cilantro sprigs

½ avocado, peeled, halved and pitted

1 cup crushed ice

¾ cup water

½ cup almond milk

2 tablespoons lime juice

1 teaspoon low-carb sweetener (Erythritol, Swerve or Stevia)

¼ teaspoon vanilla

Directions:

1. Blend all the ingredients (except for the ice) on low speed.

2. Once pureed, add ice and pulse.

3. Taste to know whether to add sweetener or lime juice.

Refreshing Anti-Inflammatory Smoothie

Prep Time: 15 minutes

Serving Size: 40g; **Serves:** 2

Ingredients:

1 celery stalk (5 to 6 inches long)

1 romaine lettuce leaf

½ cucumber, peeled and seeded

1 lime, peeled

1 pinch turmeric powder

1 teaspoon ginger powder

1 cup water

1 cup crushed ice (optional)

Directions:

1. Blend all the ingredients until smooth.

2. You may add the crushed ice if you want to consume the smoothie right away. If you plan to store and chill it for a few hours, you do not have to add the ice.

Keto Protein Shake

Prep Time: 15 minutes

Serving Size: 40g; **Serves:** 3

Ingredients:

1 egg

2 cups spinach

1 cup mixed berries (preferably raspberries, strawberries and blackberries)

¼ avocado, peeled and halved

¼ cup of water or unsweetened coconut milk

Directions:

1. Blend all the ingredients until smooth.

Dandelion Root Coffee

Prep Time: 5 minutes; **Cook Time:** 7-10 minutes

Serving Size: 40g; **Serves:** 4

Ingredients:

2 tablespoons dandelion root, ground roasted

2 tablespoons chicory root, ground roasted

4 cups water

1 cinnamon stick

heavy cream or coconut milk (optional)

Directions:

1. Put the first four ingredients in a saucepan over medium heat.

2. Bring to a boil and then allow it to simmer for 5 minutes.

3. Pour the dandelion coffee into cups or tumblers through a strainer.

4. Add heavy cream or coconut milk to sweeten.

Condiments

Keto Mayonnaise

Prep Time: 15 minutes

Net Weight: approx. 300g

Ingredients:

2 egg yolks

2 teaspoons lemon juice

1 teaspoon mustard

¾ cup coconut oil, melted

½ cup olive oil

salt and pepper

Directions:

1. Put the egg yolks, mustard and 1 teaspoon lemon juice in a blender. Blend them in the lowest setting.

2. Add the coconut oil and olive oil. Continue blending.

3. Once the oils are mixed well, add the remaining lemon juice.

4. Season it with salt and pepper before placing in a jar.

5. Refrigerate the mayonnaise. Make sure you consume it within the week.

Herb Butter

Prep Time: 10 minutes

Net Weight: approx. 145g

Ingredients:

5 ounces butter

1 garlic clove

4 tablespoons parsley

½ tablespoon garlic powder

1 teaspoon lemon juice

1 pinch salt

Directions:

1. Mix all the ingredients in one large bowl.

2. Transfer the mixture in a container and refrigerate it for at least 30 minutes before use.

Raspberry Vinaigrette

Prep Time: 15 minutes

Net Weight: approx. 380g

Ingredients:

½ cup raspberries

½ cup olive oil

½ cup white wine vinegar

35 drops Liquid Stevia

Directions:

1. Blend all the ingredients until the raspberries are no longer visible.

2. Use a strainer to separate the seeds.

3. Keep the raspberry vinaigrette in a jar.

Avocado Dressing

Prep Time: 15 minutes

Net Weight: approx. 180g

Ingredients:

1 avocado, peeled, pitted and sliced

½ cup water

3 tablespoons olive oil

1 tablespoon lemon juice

salt and pepper

Directions:

1. Put the avocado, lemon juice, olive oil and water in a blender. Blend until smooth.

2. Add a pinch of salt and pepper to season.

3. Use immediately or store in a jar.

Avocado Dip

Prep Time: 20 minutes

Net Weight: approx. 400g

Ingredients:

3 avocados, peeled, halved and pitted

1 tablespoon lemon juice

½ teaspoon chili powder

½ teaspoon salt

¼ teaspoon cumin

Directions:

1. Put the avocado meat in a bowl and mash it using a spoon.

2. Add the cumin, salt, chili and lemon juice. Stir lightly.

3. Serve immediately.

Chicken Herb Gravy

Prep Time: 1 hour; **Cook Time:** 1 hour

Net Weight: approx. 1⅛ kg

Ingredients:

1 liter chicken stock

pan drippings, either from roasted turkey or roasted chicken

2 medium onions, roughly chopped

2 garlic cloves

1 tablespoon thyme, chopped

½ teaspoon salt

Directions:

1. Cook the chicken stock, garlic and onions in a saucepan over medium heat. Bring to a boil.

2. Reduce heat to low. Allow it to simmer for about 30 minutes or until the garlic and onions are soft.

3. Add the pan drippings and mix. Remove from heat and allow it to cool.

4. Once cool, put the mixture in a blender. Blend until smooth.

5. Pour the mixture back in the saucepan. Add thyme and salt to taste.

Spicy Pesto

Prep Time: 20 minutes

Net Weight: approx.700g

Ingredients:

1½ cups basil

¾ cup parmesan cheese, grated

⅔ cup olive oil

⅓ cup pine nuts, toasted and crushed

2 teaspoons red bell pepper puree

1 teaspoon garlic, minced

salt and pepper

Directions:

1. Put all ingredients (except olive oil) in a blender. Blend for 2 minutes.

2. Add the olive oil then blend again for a minute.

3. Store the spicy pesto in a jar.

Keto Cucumber Relish

Prep Time: 10 minutes; **Cook Time:** 15-30 minutes

Net Weight: approx. 1½ kg

Ingredients:

4 cucumbers, peeled and diced

3 celery stalks, finely chopped

1 green pepper, seeded and chopped

1 red pepper, seeded and chopped

8 ounces onions, chopped

15 ounces vinegar

12 ounces Liquid Stevia (or any other low-carb sweetener)

2 ounces salt

1 tablespoon mustard seeds

Directions:

1. Put the diced cucumbers in a container.

2. Season them with the two ounces of salt.

3. Cover and set aside for at least 12 hours.

4. Use a strainer to get rid of excess water.

5. Wash the cucumbers in cold running water.

6. Put them in a pan along with the rest of the ingredients.

7. Bring the relish to a boil and let it simmer until it has thickened.

8. Store in a jar.

Keto Cucumber Pickles

Prep Time: 15 minutes

Serving Size: 150g; **Serves:** 8-10

Ingredients:

6 ounces cucumber, sliced

½ cup white vinegar

½ cup water

¼ cup Erythritol

15 drops Liquid Stevia

2 tablespoons chopped white onion

½ teaspoon cayenne pepper

½ teaspoon red pepper flakes

¼ teaspoon celery seeds

1 pinch salt

1 pinch pepper

Directions:

1. Put all the ingredients in a jar.

2. Cover and refrigerate for half a day before consuming.

Keto Pimientos

Prep Time: 15 minutes; **Cook Time:** 10 minutes

Net Weight: approx. 1¼ kg

Ingredients:

1 kilogram red peppers, seeded and halved

2½ cups vinegar

2½ cups olive oil

3 cups hot water

3 cups cold water

Directions:

1. In a large bowl, put the red peppers and pour the hot water. Wait for 2 minutes before draining the water.

2. Add the cold water, wait for 2 minutes and drain again.

3. Put the red peppers in a jar.

4. Boil the vinegar in a saucepan over medium heat.

5. Add the olive oil and bring it to a boil.

6. Add them into the jar and cover.

Blue Cheese with Keto Mayonnaise

Prep Time: 20 minutes

Net Weight: approx. 480g

Ingredients:

5 ounces blue cheese

3 parsley sprigs, finely chopped

¾ cup Greek yogurt

8 tablespoons keto mayonnaise

heavy cream

salt and pepper

Directions:

1. Tear the blue cheese into chunks.

2. Put them in a bowl and add the keto mayonnaise, Greek yogurt and parsley sprigs. Mix well.

3. Season the mixture with salt and pepper.

4. Add heavy cream to dilute.

Keto Blackberry Jam

Prep Time: 10 minutes; **Cook Time:** 25 minutes

Net Weight: approx. 500g

Ingredients:

8 ounces blackberries

30 grams chipotle peppers

8 drops Liquid Stevia

¼ cup Erythritol

¼ cup MCT oil

¼ teaspoon Guar Gum

Directions:

1. Cook the blackberries in a pan over low heat.

2. When the fruit softens, put the Liquid Stevia, Erythritol and chipotle peppers in the pan then mix. Use a spoon to crush blackberries and continue mixing.

3. Pour the MCT oil into the mixture.

4. Set the heat to medium and bring it to a boil.

5. After that, set the heat back to low and allow the mixture to simmer for at least 6 minutes.

6. Put Guar Gum and blend well.

7. Use a colander to strain the seeds before storing the blackberry jam in a jar.

Soups

Avocado Soup

Prep Time: 30 minutes; **Cook Time:** 40 minutes

Serving Size: 400g; **Serves:** 4

Ingredients:

2 avocados, peeled, halved and pitted

1½ pints chicken stock

1 tablespoon butter

2 teaspoons lemon juice

1 onion, finely chopped

salt and pepper

Directions:

1. Put the onion and chicken stock in a saucepan and let it simmer for 30 minutes.

2. While waiting, rub the avocados against a metal strainer.

3. Add the butter and lemon juice into the bowl of avocados.

4. Get the chicken stock and add the avocado mixture. Use salt and pepper to season.

Broccoli Cheese Soup

Prep Time: 30 minutes; **Cook Time:** 35-40 minutes

Serving Size: 400g; **Serves:** 4-5

Ingredients:

4 cups broccoli florets

3 cups cheddar cheese, shredded

3½ cups vegetable broth or chicken broth

4 cloves garlic, minced

1 cup heavy cream

Directions:

1. Using a large pot over medium-high heat, sauté garlic until fragrant.

2. Put the broccoli, cream and broth.

3. Set heat to high and bring it to a boil.

4. Once it boiled, set it to low heat and allow it to simmer until all the broccoli florets are tender.

5. Add the cheese ½ cup at a time.

6. Continue stirring as you put the cheese and until they all melt.

7. Remove from heat and serve in bowls.

Cauliflower Soup

Prep Time: 30 minutes; **Cook Time:** 1¼ hours

Serving Size: 400g; **Serves:** 6

Ingredients:

3 cups cauliflower florets

1½ pints chicken stock

1 garlic clove, crushed

1 onion, sliced

2 ounces butter, melted

3 tablespoons single cream

1 pinch grated nutmeg

salt and pepper

Directions:

1. Gently fry the garlic and onion in melted butter in a pot for 5 minutes.

2. Put the chicken stock and cauliflower florets. Cover the pot and bring it to boil.

3. Add salt, pepper and nutmeg. Stir for a minute.

4. Cover and let it simmer for 50 to 60 minutes.

5. Add the cream and stir well.

Chilled Asparagus Soup

Prep Time: 35 minutes; **Cook Time:** 25-30 minutes

Serving Size: 300g; **Serves:** 6

Ingredients:

16 asparagus spears

1¼ liters chicken stock

4 ounces ground almonds

salt and pepper

Directions:

1. Cut the asparagus tips and set aside.

2. Put the remainder and half the chicken stock in a blender and turn the mixture into a puree.

3. Add the puree, remaining chicken stock, and almonds in a saucepan.

4. Season the soup with salt and pepper.

5. Bring it to a boil and simmer for a minute or two.

6. Use a strainer to separate the soup and asparagus.

7. Use the asparagus as side dish.

8. Refrigerate the soup and then serve in a bowl.

9. Add the asparagus tips as garnish.

Lettuce Soup

Prep Time: 30 minutes; **Cook Time:** 20-25 minutes

Serving Size: 400g; **Serves:** 4

Ingredients:

1 lettuce, chopped

1½ pints chicken stock

1 onion, finely chopped

3 parsley sprigs, chopped

2 ounces butter

5 tablespoons single cream

1 tablespoon lemon juice

1 pinch grated nutmeg

salt and pepper

Directions:

1. Fry the onion in melted butter in a saucepan for 5 minutes.

2. Toss in the lettuce and cook for a couple of minutes.

3. Add the chicken stock and lemon juice. Season the soup with salt, pepper and nutmeg.

4. Bring it to a boil and simmer for 10 to 15 minutes.

5. Add the cream and stir well.

6. Serve in bowls. Sprinkle the chopped parsley over the soup.

Spicy Egg Drop Soup

Prep Time: 30 minutes; **Cook Time:** 10 minutes

Serving Size: 300g; **Serves:** 1

Ingredients:

1½ cups chicken broth

2 large eggs

½ cube chicken bouillon

1 tablespoon butter

1 teaspoon chili garlic paste

1 pinch keto pimientos

1 pinch chopped spring onions

Directions:

1. Put the butter, chicken broth and chicken bouillon in a pan over medium heat. Cover the pan and bring the mixture to a boil.

2. Put the chili garlic paste and mix for a minute. Turn off the heat but do not remove the pan yet.

3. Beat the eggs and add them to the chicken broth. Stir for a few times and allow the flavor to sit.

4. Garnish with the keto pimientos and spring onions before serving.

Salads

Ultimate Keto Bowl

Prep Time: 20 minutes

Serving Size: 100g; **Serves:** 6

Ingredients:

1 avocado, peeled, pitted and chopped

1 lettuce, shredded

450 grams asparagus tips

400 grams artichoke hearts

3 green olives, chopped

4 tablespoons raspberry vinaigrette

Directions:

1. Mix all the ingredients (except for the raspberry vinaigrette) in a bowl.

2. Add the raspberry vinaigrette and mix until all the avocados and vegetables are coated.

Green Cleanse Salad

Prep Time: 25 minutes

Serving Size: 150g; **Serves:** 4

Ingredients:

2 cucumbers, peeled and spiralized

½ avocado, peeled, pitted and sliced length-wise

½ cup broccoli florets

¼ cup celery, chopped

⅛ cup pistachios, crushed

2 tablespoons lemon juice

1 tablespoon olive oil

salt and pepper

Directions:

1. Put the avocado slices in a bowl.

2. Add the olive oil, lemon juice, salt and pepper.

3. Mash the mixture using a fork.

4. Toss in the rest of the ingredients and mix well.

Mixed Greens Salad

Prep Time: 15 minutes

Serving Size: 150g; **Serves:** 2

Ingredients:

2 ounces green leafy vegetables (preferably kale, spinach, lettuce and Swiss chard)

3 tablespoons roasted pine nuts

2 tablespoons parmesan cheese, shaved

2 tablespoons raspberry vinaigrette

salt and pepper

Directions:

1. Mix all the ingredients until most of the greens are coated with the raspberry vinaigrette.

Spinach Avocado Strawberry Salad

Prep Time: 20 minutes

Serving Size: 150g; **Serves:** 5

Ingredients:

6 cups young spinach

2 avocados, peeled, pitted and diced

1 pint strawberries, sliced

¼ cup almonds, sliced and toasted

4 ounces blue cheese, crumbled

½ red onion, sliced

raspberry vinaigrette

Directions:

1. Mix all the ingredients (except for the raspberry vinaigrette) in a bowl.

2. Pour your desired amount of raspberry vinaigrette over the mixture.

Spinach and Mushroom Salad

Prep Time: 30 minutes

Serving Size: 150g; **Serves:** 4

Ingredients:

½ kilogram spinach, washed and dried

12 ounces mushrooms, finely chopped

3 parsley sprigs, finely chopped

2 spring onions, finely chopped

1 garlic clove, crushed

4 tablespoons olive oil

1 tablespoon lemon juice

raspberry vinaigrette

salt and pepper

Directions:

1. Tear the spinach leaves.

2. Mix the leaves, mushrooms and spring onions in a salad bowl.

3. In another bowl, put the remaining ingredients (except the parsley sprigs) and toss well. This serves as the dressing for the salad.

4. Pour the dressing over the spinach, mushrooms and spring onions.

5. Garnish with the chopped parsley sprigs before serving.

Cucumber Salad

Prep Time: 20 minutes

Serving Size: 100g; **Serves:** 4

Ingredients:

2 cucumbers, thinly sliced

1 onion, chopped

3 tablespoons vinegar

1 teaspoon low-carb sweetener (Erythritol, Swerve or Stevia)

¼ teaspoon white pepper

1 tablespoon water

Directions:

1. Mix all the ingredients in a salad bowl until the cucumber slices are well-coated.

2. Refrigerate for 30 minutes.

3. Strain to get rid of the excess liquid before serving.

Cottage Cheese and Berry Salad

Prep Time: 20 minutes

Serving Size: 150g; **Serves:** 4

Ingredients:

12 ounces cottage cheese

1½ cups mixed berries (preferably raspberries, blackberries and strawberries)

1 ounce nuts, chopped

6 lettuce leaves

Directions:

1. Put the berries, nuts and cheese in a bowl and mix well.

2. Arrange the lettuce leaves in a salad bowl.

3. Fill the lettuce lined salad bowl with the cheese and berry mixture in the center.

4. Serve as it is or drizzle over your favorite keto salad dressing.

Beef

Roasted Beef Fillet

Prep Time: 20 minutes**; Cook Time:** 30 minutes

Serving Size: 150g; **Serves:** 6

Ingredients:

1½ kilograms beef fillet

125 grams butter, melted

salt and pepper

½ cup water

Directions:

1. Preheat oven to 425 degrees Fahrenheit.

2. Season the beef fillet with salt and pepper and place it on the roasting pan.

3. Pour the melted butter over the beef fillet.

4. Put the pan into the preheated oven and roast for 5 minutes. Lower down the temperature into 350 degrees Fahrenheit and bake for a further 20 minutes.

5. Transfer the roasted beef fillet in a serving plate and put it back in the oven for 10 minutes. No need to turn the oven on again.

6. Gather the juices from the roasting pan into a skillet and add the water. Bring it to a boil.

7. Slice the roasted beef fillet to your preferred thickness. Pour the juices over the meat.

Jalapeño Cheddar Burger

Prep Time: 15 minutes; **Cook Time:** 12 minutes

Serving Size: 150g; **Serves:** 3-4

Ingredients:

28 ounces lean beef (may be replaced with turkey)

1 jalapeño pepper, diced

2 ounces cheddar cheese, shredded

4 tablespoons cream cheese

2 tablespoons onion, minced

¼ teaspoon garlic powder

salt and pepper

olive oil

Directions:

1. Preheat grill to medium heat.

2. Mix the diced jalapeño pepper, cheddar cheese, cream cheese and garlic powder in one bowl.

3. Take the lean meat and season it with salt, pepper and onion.

4. Cut the meat into four equal pieces.

5. Get ¼ of the jalapeño mixture and flatten it in your desired shape. This will serve as the filling for the burger.

6. Get a piece of meat and use it to wrap the jalapeño mixture.

7. Coat the burgers with olive oil. Put the burgers in the preheated grill

8. Grill for 6 minutes for each side before flipping over to cook the other side.

Keto Sweet and Sour Meatballs

Prep Time: 30 minutes; **Cook Time:** 20 minutes

Serving Size: 150g; **Serves:** 6

Ingredients:

1 pound ground beef

1 egg

1½ cups water

1 cup Erythritol

⅓ cup sugar-free ketchup

¼ cup Parmesan cheese, grated

¼ cup apple cider vinegar

½ teaspoon xanthan gum

¼ teaspoon onion powder

Directions:

1. Mix the ground beef, Parmesan cheese, onion powder and 1 egg in one large bowl using your hands.

2. Get a spoonful of the mixture and mold it into small balls. You can make around 30 meatballs with the mixture.

3. Place the meatballs in a preheated saucepan and cook under medium heat until it is mostly brown.

4. Take them out of the saucepan and set aside as you make the sauce.

5. Using the same saucepan, put the water, Erythritol, ketchup and vinegar. Mix them using a whisk.

6. Add the xanthan gum into the saucepan as you mix.

7. When the mixture thickens, set the heat to low and allow it to simmer.

8. After 2 to 3 minutes, add the meatballs and let it simmer until they are completely cooked.

Keto Beef Stroganoff

Prep Time: 20 minutes; **Cook Time:** 15 minutes

Serving Size: 150g; **Serves:** 6

Ingredients:

1 kilogram beef, thinly sliced

8 ounces mushroom, sliced

1 onion, chopped

3 parsley sprigs, finely chopped

5 ounces sour cream

2 ounces butter

salt and pepper

Directions:

1. Melt the 2 ounces of butter in a pan over medium heat.

2. Put the chopped onion and gently fry until fragrant.

3. Add the beef slices and cook for 8 minutes.

4. Put the mushrooms and stir occasionally. Cook the mushrooms for a further 3 minutes.

5. Add the cream and season the dish with salt and pepper.

6. Transfer to a serving dish and use the parsley sprigs to garnish.

Beef with Zucchini

Prep Time: 15 minutes; **Cook Time:** 10 minutes

Serving Size: 150g; **Serves:** 2-3

Ingredients:

300 grams beef, sliced into strips

1 zucchini, sliced into long thin strips

3 garlic cloves, minced

¼ cup cilantro, chopped

2 tablespoons tamari sauce

olive oil

Directions:

1. Heat two tablespoons of olive oil in a pan over medium heat.

2. Add the beef strips and sauté for a few minutes with the heat set to high.

3. Put the zucchini slices once the beef strips turn brown. Sauté the zucchini slices.

4. Add the cilantro, garlic and tamari sauce and then sauté.

5. Transfer to a serving dish.

Beef in Lettuce Wraps

Prep Time: 35 minutes; **Cook Time:** 20-25 minutes

Serving Size: 150g; **Serves:** 6

Ingredients:

2 pounds ground beef (may be replaced with ground pork or chicken)

2 cups beef broth (replace with chicken broth if using pork or chicken)

1 bunch of cilantro, finely chopped

1 bunch of mint, finely chopped

1 romaine lettuce

3 garlic cloves, crushed

⅓ cup lime juice

3 tablespoons fish sauce

salt

Directions:

1. Cook the ground meat in a skillet over medium heat for 8 to 10 minutes. Use a spatula to break them apart and to cook them evenly.

2. Pour the beef broth over the ground beef. Add a pinch of salt to season.

3. Stir occasionally and allow it to simmer for 6 to 8 minutes, or until the beef broth boiled off.

4. While you wait, mix the fish sauce, lime juice and crushed garlic.

5. Combine the chopped cilantro and mint in another bowl.

6. Tear each lettuce leaf, place in a plate and set aside.

7. When the beef broth completely boiled away, add the lime juice mixture and let it simmer for 2 to 3 minutes.

8. Add the mint and cilantro. Stir for a minute before removing the beef from heat.

9. Spoon the beef into each lettuce leaf.

10. Arrange the beef filled leaves in a serving dish.

Pork

Keto Pork Bites

Prep Time: 15 minutes; **Cook Time:** 30-45 minutes

Serving Size: 100g; **Serves:** 3-4

Ingredients:

10.5 ounces pork (preferably belly strips for crispier pork bites)

1.76 ounces blue cheese

¼ large onion, diced

4 tablespoons heavy cream

1 tablespoon butter

salt and pepper

Directions:

1. Preheat oven to 480 degrees Fahrenheit.

2. Slice the pork into strips and rub it with salt before placing them into the baking sheet.

3. Bake for 30 to 45 minutes. The pork slices should have crispy brown color before you take them out.

4. While you wait, make the sauce by putting the butter and onion in a pan over medium heat.

5. Add the heavy cream once the onion caramelized.

6. After a minute, add the blue cheese and let it melt.

7. When the cheese melted, set heat to high for a couple of minutes.

8. Remove from heat and let it cool.

9. Take out the baked pork slices and transfer them into a serving plate.

10. Pour over the sauce or serve it in a bowl.

Pork and Liver Pâté

Prep Time: 20 minutes; **Cook Time:** 1½ hours

Serving Size: 150g; **Serves:** 6

Ingredients:

1½ pounds pork belly, diced

8 ounces pig's liver, chopped

1 ounce butter, melted

1 onion, chopped

1 garlic clove, minced

salt and pepper

Directions:

1. Preheat oven to 300 degrees Fahrenheit.

2. Put the pork, liver, garlic and onion in a cutting board. Mix and chop them together at least three times. Season the mixture with salt and pepper.

3. Put the mixture in an ovenproof dish with a dedicated lid. Cover with foil before putting on the lid.

4. Fill half of the roasting pan with water and then place the dish for the covered pork and liver mixture in the middle of the pan.

5. Put the roasting pan in the preheated oven and wait for 1½ hours before taking the dish out.

6. Remove the ovenproof lid and let the pâté cool.

7. When it is cooled completely, pour over the butter and refrigerate.

Crispy Pork Leg

Prep Time: 15 minutes; **Cook Time:** 45 minutes

Serving Size: 150g; **Serves:** 6

Ingredients:

2 kilograms pork leg, scored

¼ cup olive oil

ground ginger

salt

Directions:

1. Preheat oven to 425 degrees Fahrenheit.

2. Spread the olive oil on a roasting pan.

3. Rub the pork leg with the ginger and salt. Use more salt if you want the pork leg to be extra crispy.

4. Put the pork leg in the pan. Place the pan in the preheated oven and roast for 20 minutes.

5. Set the temperature down to 350 degrees Fahrenheit and roast for a further 25 minutes or until the pork leg is browned.

6. Transfer in a serving plate.

Poultry

Chicken with Herb Butter

Prep Time: 10 minutes; **Cook Time:** 8-10 minutes

Serving Size: 150g; **Serves:** 2

Ingredients:

4 chicken breasts

1 ounce butter

salt and pepper

herb butter

Directions:

1. Rub the chicken breasts with salt and pepper.

2. Melt the butter in a pan over medium heat.

3. Put the seasoned chicken breasts and fry until fully cooked.

4. Spread herb butter on the fried chicken breasts before serving.

Chicken Pad Thai

Prep Time: 35 minutes; **Cook Time:** 10 minutes

Serving Size: 150g; **Serves:** 4

Ingredients:

2 pounds chicken tenders

3 eggs, beaten

⅓ cup chicken broth

4 zucchini, spiralized

2 garlic cloves, minced

½ cup spring onions, chopped

3 tablespoons peanut butter

2 tablespoons peanut oil

½ cup crushed peanuts

1 tablespoon vinegar

2 tablespoons tamari

1 teaspoon red pepper flakes

1 pinch garlic powder

1 pinch ground ginger

salt and pepper

Directions:

1. Mix garlic powder, ginger, salt and pepper in one bowl.

2. Add the chicken tenders and coat it with the mixture.

3. Pour the peanut oil in a skillet over medium heat.

4. Once the oil is hot, put the chicken tenders in the skillet and cook for about 3 minutes.

5. Get the chicken, slice it thinly, and set aside in a plate.

6. Put the beaten eggs in the skillet and scramble.

7. Remove the eggs after a minute and set them aside in another plate.

8. From medium, set the heat into low.

9. Add the vinegar, tamari, chicken broth, garlic, spring onion, peanut butter, and red pepper flakes and stir for 3 minutes.

10. Put the chicken slices, scrambled eggs and spiralized zucchini in the skillet. Mix well for a minute.

11. Garnish the Chicken Pad Thai with crushed peanuts before serving.

Keto Chicken Burger

Prep Time: 15 minutes; **Cook Time:** 6-10 minutes

Serving Size: 150g; **Serves:** 4-6

Ingredients:

1 kilogram chicken, minced

2 eggs

2 garlic cloves, finely chopped

½ onion, finely chopped

¼ cup coriander, chopped

3 tablespoons lime juice

4 tablespoons olive oil

1 teaspoon grated ginger

salt

Directions:

1. Put all the ingredients in one bowl and mix them by hand.

2. Scoop 2 tablespoons of the mixture and form it into a ball.

3. Flatten it out in a plate. Repeat the steps 2 and 3 for the rest of the mixture.

4. Heat 1 tablespoon of olive oil in a frying pan over medium heat.

5. Place the chicken patties and cook each side for 3 to 5 minutes before flipping over.

6. Refer to the condiments section to make the spread for your chicken burgers.

Creamy Chicken Casserole

Prep Time: 25 minutes; **Cook Time:** 35 minutes

Serving Size: 150g; **Serves:** 4

Ingredients:

2 pounds chicken thighs

⅔ pound cauliflower florets, washed and dried

7 ounces cheese, shredded

1¼ cups whipping cream

1 leek, chopped

3 tablespoons butter

2 tablespoons keto pesto

2 tablespoons lemon juice

salt and pepper

Directions:

1. Preheat oven to 400 degrees Fahrenheit.

2. Put the cream, keto pesto, lemon juice, salt and pepper in a bowl. Mix well.

3. Rub salt and pepper to the chicken thighs.

4. Melt the butter in a frying pan over medium heat.

5. Put the chicken thighs in the pan and fry for 5 minutes or until they turn golden brown.

6. Place the fried chicken thighs in a baking dish.

7. Sprinkle the cauliflower florets, chopped leek and shredded cheese over the chicken thighs.

8. Bake for 30 minutes.

Keto Garlic Chicken

Prep Time: 15 minutes; **Cook Time:** 30-40 minutes

Serving Size: 150g; **Serves:** 4

Ingredients:

1 kilogram chicken thighs

8 garlic cloves, sliced

8 tablespoons chopped parsley

4 tablespoons butter, melted

3 lemon juice

2 tablespoons olive oil

Directions:

1. Preheat oven to 450 degrees Fahrenheit.

2. Evenly spread the melted butter in a baking pan.

3. Season the chicken thighs with salt and pepper, and put them in the baking pan.

4. Drizzle the olive oil and lemon juice over the meat. Sprinkle the parsley and garlic as well.

5. Put the pan in the preheated oven and bake for 30 to 40 minutes. Reduce the temperature towards the last few minutes.

6. Transfer to a serving dish.

Grilled Chicken with Avocado and Strawberry

Prep Time: 20 minutes; **Cook Time:** 10 minutes

Serving Size: 150g; **Serves:** 2

Ingredients:

2 chicken breasts

1 avocado, peeled, pitted and diced

1 cup strawberries, chopped

1 jalapeño, diced

1 small onion, chopped

1 bunch of cilantro, chopped

3 tablespoons lime juice

salt and pepper

Directions:

1. Season the chicken breasts with salt and pepper. Set aside in a bowl.

2. In another bowl, mix the avocado, strawberries, jalapeño, onion, cilantro and lime. Add salt to taste. Mix well and set aside.

3. Get the chicken breasts and grill over medium heat for 5 minutes. Flip over and grill the other side for a further 5 minutes.

4. Transfer the grilled chicken to a serving dish and top with the avocado and strawberry mixture.

Chicken Celery Sticks

Prep Time: 30 minutes

Serving Size: 150g; **Serves:** 3

Ingredients:

2 cups chicken, shredded

6 celery stalks, halved

2 chives, finely chopped

¼ cup keto mayonnaise

½ teaspoon garlic powder

salt and pepper

Directions:

1. Except for the celery stalks and chives, put all the ingredients in a bowl and mix them.

2. Use the chicken mixture as a filling for the celery stalks.

3. Serve with the chopped chives as garnish.

Chicken with Basil

Prep Time: 20 minutes; **Cook Time:** 10 minutes

Serving Size: 150g; **Serves:** 2

Ingredients:

2 cups chicken breast, chopped

¼ cup basil leaves, chopped

3 garlic cloves, chopped

2 tablespoons olive oil

2 tablespoons chili, minced

2 teaspoons fish sauce

1 teaspoon ginger, minced

1 teaspoon low-carb sweetener (Erythritol, Swerve or Stevia)

Directions:

1. Heat the olive oil in a pan.

2. Put the ginger, garlic and chili. Sauté for a couple of minutes.

3. Put the chicken and cook for 5 minutes.

4. Add the basil leaves, sweetener and fish sauce. Stir and cook for 3 minutes.

5. Transfer to a serving plate.

Creamy and Cheesy Turkey

Prep Time: 20 minutes; **Cook Time:** 25-30 minutes

Serving Size: 150g; **Serves:** 4

Ingredients:

1⅓ pounds turkey breast

2 cups heavy cream

7 ounces cream cheese

7 tablespoons small capers

2 tablespoons butter

salt and pepper

Directions:

1. Preheat oven to 350 degrees Fahrenheit.

2. Melt 1 tablespoon of butter in a large ovenproof pan over medium heat. Sprinkle salt and pepper over the pan.

3. Add the turkey breast and gently fry for 5 minutes or until golden brown.

4. Put the turkey in the preheated oven and bake until the meat is completely cooked.

5. Transfer the meat in a plate and cover with foil.

6. Get the excess oil from the ovenproof pan and put them in another pan over medium heat.

7. Add the heavy cream, cream cheese, salt and pepper. Stir the mixture and bring it to a boil.

8. Set heat to low and allow it to simmer until the mixture thickens.

9. Take another pan and melt the remaining 1 tablespoon of butter.

10. Put the capers in the pan and sauté until crispy.

11. Transfer the turkey in a serving dish.

12. Pour over the cream and cheese mixture.

13. Place the crispy capers beside the turkey.

Eggs

Spinach Stuffed Eggs

Prep Time: 30 minutes

Serving Size: 80g; **Serves:** 4

Ingredients:

4 eggs, hard-boiled and halved

2 tablespoons cooked spinach, chopped

2 tablespoons parmesan cheese, grated

2 ounces cream cheese

1 pinch grated nutmeg

1 pinch cayenne pepper

salt and pepper

Directions:

1. Put the parmesan cheese, cream cheese and chopped spinach in a mixing bowl.

2. Get the yolks from the eggs and toss it the bowl as well. Mix until smooth.

3. Season the mixture with nutmeg, salt and pepper.

4. Stuff the spinach and cheese mix into the egg whites.

5. Sprinkle the cayenne pepper over the eggs before serving.

Salmon Stuffed Eggs

Prep Time: 30 minutes

Serving Size: 80g; **Serves:** 4

Ingredients:

4 eggs, hard-boiled and halved

2 ounces salmon, grilled and chopped

8 lettuce leaves

1 teaspoon lemon juice

½ ounce butter, softened

salt and pepper

Directions:

1. Get the yolks from the eggs and put them in a bowl.

2. Add the salmon, lemon juice, butter, salt and pepper.

3. Mix well and stuff them into the egg whites.

4. Get 4 serving plates. Put two lettuce leaves in one plate. Put two salmon-stuffed egg whites on the lettuce leaves.

Egg Salad in Avocados

Prep Time: 20 minutes

Serving Size: 150g; Serves: 6

Ingredients:

6 large eggs, hard boiled and chopped

3 medium avocados, peeled, halved and pitted

3 ribs celery, chopped

⅓ medium red onion, chopped

4 tablespoons keto mayonnaise

2 tablespoons lime juice

2 teaspoons brown mustard

1 teaspoon hot sauce

½ teaspoon cumin

salt and pepper

Directions:

1. Mix all the ingredients except for the avocadoes.

2. Spoon the egg salad mixture into the avocado halves.

Offal

Chopped Chicken Livers on Lettuce Leaves

Prep Time: 20 minutes; **Cook Time:** 5 minutes

Serving Size: 80g; **Serves:** 8

Ingredients:

½ kilogram chicken livers

50 grams chicken fat

8 lettuce leaves

1 onion, finely chopped

2 eggs, hard-boiled and chopped

1 egg yolk, sieved

salt and pepper

Directions:

1. Melt chicken fat in a pan over low heat.

2. Add the onion and gently fry.

3. Put the chicken livers and cook for 2 to 3 minutes.

4. Set aside to cool and then chop the livers.

5. Mix the chopped chicken livers, hard-boiled eggs and onion in a bowl. Season the mixture with salt and pepper.

6. Get eight serving plates and put one lettuce leaf on each.

7. Scoop the liver and egg mixture and put them on the lettuce leaves.

8. Toss the egg yolk over the eight servings.

Chicken Liver Pâté

Prep Time: 25 minutes; **Cook Time:** 6-8 minutes

Serving Size: 80g; **Serves:** 8

Ingredients:

½ kilogram chicken livers, chopped

2 garlic cloves, crushed

2 onions, finely chopped

2 parsley sprigs, chopped

6 ounces butter

1 bay leaf

1 pinch thyme

salt and pepper

Directions:

1. Melt 4 ounces of butter in a pan over medium heat.

2. Toss in the garlic and onion and fry until soft.

3. Put the chopped chicken livers in the pan and fry for three more minutes.

4. Add salt, pepper, parsley, thyme and bay leaf to taste. Mix for two minutes.

5. Remove from heat, get the bay leaf and leave the mixture to cool.

6. Once cool, pour the mixture into the blender and blend until pureed.

7. Melt 2 ounces of butter and add it to the pureed mixture.

8. Transfer to a foil lined container and cover with a lid.

9. Refrigerate before serving.

Chicken Liver with Thyme Butter

Prep Time: 30 minutes; **Cook Time:** 8-10 minutes

Serving Size: 100g; **Serves:** 4

Ingredients:

1 pound chicken liver

1 garlic clove, finely chopped

1 red onion, finely chopped

10 ounces butter

1 tablespoon dried thyme

1 tablespoon tomato paste

1 teaspoon black pepper

Directions:

1. Melt 2 ounces of butter in a pan over medium heat.

2. Put the garlic and onion and then gently fry.

3. Transfer to a small bowl.

4. Set heat to high. Put additional 2 ounces of butter in the pan.

5. Add the chicken livers and fry until all sides are cooked. Sprinkle salt and pepper to taste.

6. Reduce heat and scoop out some of the melted butter.

7. Transfer the fried livers in a plate and allow it to cool for at least 2 minutes.

8. Put the fried livers, garlic and onion in a blender or food processor. Add the tomato paste and 4 ounces of butter. Blend until smooth.

9. Put the mixture evenly in a baking dish.

10. In another pan, melt 4 ounces of butter.

11. Transfer the melted butter in a bowl. Add the pepper and thyme. Stir well.

12. Pour the thyme butter over the liver, garlic and onion mix.

13. Refrigerate for at least an hour before serving.

Lemon Garlic Kidneys

Prep Time: 15 minutes; **Cook Time:** 15 minutes

Serving Size: 150g; **Serves:** 4

Ingredients:

8 lamb kidneys, sliced

3 tablespoons lemon juice

2 garlic cloves, crushed

2 ounces butter

salt and pepper

Directions:

1. Coat the kidneys with salt and pepper.

2. Melt the butter in a pan over medium heat.

3. Toss in the garlic and kidney slices.

4. Fry until all sides of the kidney slices are brown.

5. Add the lemon juice and continue to fry for 10 minutes.

Fish

Wild Salmon with Keto Pesto

Prep Time: 10 minutes; **Cook Time:** 8-10 minutes

Serving Size: 150g; **Serves:** 3-4

Ingredients:

4 to 6 ounces of wild salmon

½ cup keto pesto

olive oil

salt

Directions:

1. Clean the wild salmon and sprinkle salt over the fish.

2. Heat olive oil in the grill pan over medium heat.

3. Cook each side for 4 to 5 minutes.

4. Put the cooked wild salmon in paper towels to get rid of excess oil.

5. Place the fish in a serving dish.

6. Pour over the keto pesto before serving.

Baked Salmon Fillets

Prep Time: 20 minutes; **Cook Time:** 25 minutes

Serving Size: 150g; **Serves:** 2

Ingredients:

½ kilogram salmon fillets

2 to 3 tablespoons lemon juice

paprika

salt and pepper

Directions:

1. Preheat oven to 375 degrees Fahrenheit.

2. Season the salmon fillets with paprika, salt and pepper.

3. Add the lemon juice and make sure all the fillets are coated.

4. Place the seasoned salmon fillets in a foil lined baking sheet.

5. Put the baking sheet in the preheated oven and bake for 25 minutes.

Foil-Baked Salmon Fillets with Asparagus

Prep Time: 30 minutes; **Cook Time:** 10-12 minutes

Serving Size: 150g; **Serves:** 4

Ingredients:

2 wild salmon fillets (about 8 ounces)

16 asparagus spears

3 parsley sprigs, chopped

4 lemon slices

4 onion slices

1 tablespoon olive oil

1 teaspoon dried oregano

salt and pepper

Directions:

1. Preheat oven to 400 degrees Fahrenheit.

2. In a bowl, season the wild salmon fillets with salt, pepper, oregano and olive oil.

3. Get 2 foil sheets. Arrange 8 asparagus spears in one sheet and the remaining asparagus spears in the other sheet.

4. Place the seasoned wild salmon fillets over the asparagus spears.

5. Put 2 onion slices and 2 lemon slices at the top of each wild salmon fillet.

6. Wrap the foil and put them in a baking sheet.

7. Bake for 10 to 12 minutes. Do not go beyond 12 minutes as the asparagus spears might become too soft.

8. Gently open the foil.

9. Get a spatula and carefully transfer the baked salmon in a serving dish.

10. Use the parsley sprigs to garnish.

Baked Sea Bass with Herbs and Cauliflowers

Prep Time: 30 minutes; **Cook Time:** 15 minutes

Serving Size: 150g; **Serves:** 2

Ingredients:

1 whole sea bass, scaled and cleaned

1 cup cauliflower, grated

⅓ cup fresh mint, chopped

⅓ cup parsley, chopped

⅓ cup green olives

3 tablespoons olive oil

2 small lemons

salt and pepper

Directions:

1. Preheat oven to 400 degrees Fahrenheit.

2. Rub 1 tablespoon of olive oil around the sea bass and season it using salt and pepper.

3. Insert two slices of lemon and half of the mint and parsley into the fish.

4. Place the fish on a parchment paper lined baking pan and put it in the preheated oven for 15 minutes.

5. While waiting, juice the remaining lemon and slice the olives.

6. Mix the olives, cauliflower, lemon juice, 2 tablespoons of olive oil and the remaining herbs in a bowl.

7. Put a bit of salt and pepper into the mixture.

8. Take out the sea bass from the oven and put it in a serving plate.

9. Slowly pour the cauliflower and herb mixture over the sea bass.

Grilled Mackerel Pâté

Prep Time: 30 minutes

Serving Size: 80g; **Serves:** 6

Ingredients:

2 mackerels, grilled, skinned and boned

10 ounces butter, softened

3 ounces cream cheese

3 parsley sprigs, chopped

5 teaspoons lemon juice

salt and pepper

Directions:

1. Mix and mash the mackerel and butter using a fork.

2. Add the lemon juice and cream cheese gradually as you mix.

3. Season the mixture with salt and pepper.

4. Refrigerate for an hour and then use the chopped parsley to garnish.

Grilled Trout Pâté

Prep Time: 30 minutes

Serving Size: 80g; **Serves:** 6

Ingredients:

2 trout, grilled, skinned and boned

3 ounces heavy cream

8 ounces butter, softened

3 parsley sprigs, chopped

2 tablespoons lemon juice

salt and pepper

Directions:

1. Mix and mash the trout and butter in a bowl using a fork.

2. Add the lemon juice and cream gradually as you mix.

3. Add salt and pepper to taste.

4. Refrigerate for an hour. Use the chopped parsley to garnish.

Buttered Trout and Shrimp

Prep Time: 30-40 minutes; **Cook Time:** 15 minutes

Serving Size: 150g; **Serves:** 4

Ingredients:

4 trout, cleaned

4 ounces small shrimps, peeled and deveined

4 ounces mushrooms, sliced

5 ounces butter

2 tablespoons lemon juice

Directions:

1. Melt the 5 ounces of butter in a pan over medium heat.

2. Put the trout and fry for 10 minutes or until their flesh flakes easily.

3. Remove the fried trout and set aside in a serving plate.

4. Fry the shrimps and mushrooms in the pan for 5 minutes.

5. Add the lemon juice and mix.

6. Pour the mixture over the fried trout.

Buttered Trout with Almonds

Prep Time: 30 minutes; **Cook Time:** 13 minutes

Serving Size: 150g; **Serves:** 4

Ingredients:

4 trout, cleaned

4 olives

3 ounces butter

2 ounces almonds

salt and pepper

parsley sprigs

Directions:

1. Melt 1½ ounce of butter in a pan over medium heat.

2. Put the almonds and fry for 5 minutes or until golden brown.

3. Get the toasted almonds and place them in a plate.

4. Put the remaining butter in the pan and melt.

5. Put the 4 trout and fry for at least 8 minutes or until the skin and flesh flake easily. Add salt and pepper to taste.

6. Transfer the fried fish in a serving dish.

7. Insert one olive in the mouth of each trout.

8. Get the melted butter in the pan and pour over the fried fish.

9. Add the almonds and parsley sprigs to garnish.

Buttered Hake Cutlets with Almonds and Mushrooms

Prep Time: 30 minutes; **Cook Time:** 13 minutes

Serving Size: 150g; **Serves:** 4-6

Ingredients:

4 hakes, sliced into cutlets

4 ounces mushrooms, sliced

3 ounces blanched almonds

2 ounces butter, melted

1 ounce butter

1 ounce parmesan cheese, shredded

salt and pepper

Directions:

1. Wash the hake cutlets and rub them with pepper and salt.

2. Place them on the grill rack or pan.

3. Spread the 1 ounce of melted butter and put half of the shredded parmesan cheese over the cutlets.

4. Grill for at least 5 minutes or until both the skin and the flesh are brown.

5. Flip over Hand spread the remaining butter and sprinkle the remaining parmesan cheese.

6. Cook for another 5 minutes or until brown. Set aside to cool.

7. Melt the 1 ounce of butter in a pan over medium heat.

8. Put the almonds and mushrooms in the pan and fry for at least 3 minutes.

9. Pour the mushroom and almond mix over the hake cutlets in a serving dish.

Grilled Haddock Pâté

Prep Time: 30 minutes

Serving Size: 100g; **Serves:** 4

Ingredients:

4 ounces haddock, grilled, skinned and boned

1 shallot, finely chopped

4 ounces butter

1 teaspoon lemon juice

3 parsley sprigs, finely chopped

1 pinch garlic powder

pepper

Directions:

1. Put the haddock and butter in a bowl and mash them together using a fork.

2. Add the remaining ingredients (except the chopped parsley sprigs) in the bowl and mix well.

3. Season the mixture with pepper.

4. Refrigerate for at least an hour and then serve with the parsley sprigs as garnish.

Seafood

Steamed Clams with Melted Butter

Prep Time: 30 minutes; **Cook Time:** 30-40 minutes

Serving Size: 150g ; **Serves:** 4-6

Ingredients:

6 pints clams

4 ounces butter, melted

salt and pepper

Directions:

1. Inspect the clams and toss out the ones that have holes or are slightly opened.

2. Scrub the clams to get rid of dirt and blemishes.

3. Wash them using cold running water.

4. Fill a large saucepan with ½ inch layer of water with 1 tablespoon salt.

5. Put the clams in the saucepan, cover and steam until all or most of the clams open.

6. Arrange the opened clams in a serving plate.

7. Pour the melted butter over the clams.

Spicy Shrimp and Pork Bites

Prep Time: 40 minutes; **Cook Time:** 35-40 minutes

Serving Size: 150g; **Serves:** 4

Ingredients:

1 pound shrimp, peeled and deveined

1 pound ground pork

4 stalks spring onion, finely chopped

3 green bell peppers

2 red bell peppers

1 large egg

1 tablespoon minced garlic

1 tablespoon sesame oil

2 teaspoons fish sauce

1 teaspoon vinegar

salt and pepper

Directions:

1. Put all of the ingredients (except the bell peppers) in one big Ziploc bag and mix well. Open the bag to get rid of excess air. Refrigerate for at least a couple of hours.

2. Preheat oven to 375 degrees Fahrenheit.

3. As you wait, slice the stems of the bell peppers and cut them into quarters. Remove the seeds and membranes.

4. Fill each pepper quarter with the shrimp and pork mixture.

5. Arrange them in a parchment paper lined baking sheet and put in the preheated oven. Bake for 35 to 40 minutes.

6. Take the baking sheet out and leave the baked shrimp and pork bites to cool for at least five minutes before serving.

Shrimp with Cucumber Salad

Prep Time: 20 minutes; **Cook Time:** 5-6 minutes

Serving Size: 120g; **Serves:** 2-3

Ingredients:

1 pound shrimp, peeled and deveined

3 tablespoons olive oil

2 cups cucumber salad

Directions:

1. Put 2 tablespoons of olive oil in a pan over medium heat.

2. Allow the oil to heat.

3. Put the shrimps and cook for 3 minutes.

4. Place the cucumber salad in a bowl and add the cooked shrimps.

5. Mix well and drizzle the remaining olive oil before serving.

Lobster with Keto Mayonnaise

Prep Time: 40 minutes

Serving Size: 100g; **Serves:** 4

Ingredients:

1½ pounds lobster, cooked

10 fluid ounces keto mayonnaise

6 parsley sprigs, finely chopped

3 tablespoons double cream

2 tablespoons lemon juice

salt and pepper

Directions:

1. Get the lobster meat and slice into bite-sized pieces.

2. Keep the shells in a container.

3. Put the lobster meat and the rest of the ingredients in a bowl. Mix well.

4. Take the shells and fill them with the lobster meat mixture.

Vegetables

Cheesy Zucchini Gratin

Prep Time: 30 minutes; **Cook Time:** 46 minutes

Serving Size: 100g; **Serves:** 4

Ingredients:

4 cups zucchini, sliced

1 onion, sliced

1½ cups pepper jack cheese, shredded

½ cup whipping cream

2 tablespoons butter

½ teaspoon garlic powder

olive oil

salt and pepper

Directions:

1. Preheat oven to 375 degrees Fahrenheit.

2. Mix zucchini and onion slices in one bowl.

3. Pour olive oil on your pan and fill it with ⅓ of the zucchini and onion mixture.

4. Sprinkle the shredded cheese, salt and pepper over the mixture. Put more layers until you have placed all the slices and shredded cheese.

5. In a microwave-safe dish, mix the whipping cream, garlic powder and butter. Put in the microwave for a full minute and stir.

6. Pour it over the layers of zucchini.

7. Place it inside the preheated oven and bake for 45 minutes.

Zucchini Lasagna

Prep Time: 10 minutes; **Cook Time:** 3-5 minutes

Serving Size: 80g; **Serves:** 1

Ingredients:

⅓ zucchini, spiralized

3 ounces mozzarella

3 tablespoons marinara

2 tablespoons ricotta

oregano (optional)

Directions:

1. Get a microwave-safe mug or bowl and spread 1 tablespoon of marinara on it.

2. Put a layer of the zucchini slices.

3. Top the zucchini with ricotta and another tablespoon of marinara.

4. Place the mozzarella at the top.

5. Heat it in the microwave for 3 to 5 minutes.

6. Put oregano over the lasagna if you like.

Chicken Stuffed Zucchini Boats

Prep Time: 35-40 minutes; **Cook Time:** 35 minutes

Serving Size: 80g; **Serves:** 4

Ingredients:

6 ounces rotisserie chicken

2 large zucchinis, halved and seeded

1 cup broccoli florets

1 stalk spring onion

3 ounces cheddar cheese, shredded

4 tablespoons butter, melted

2 tablespoons sour cream

salt and pepper

Directions:

1. Preheat oven to 400 degrees Fahrenheit.

2. Put 1 tablespoon of melted butter in each zucchini half. Sprinkle salt and pepper as well.

3. Arrange the four zucchini boats in a parchment paper lined baking sheet.

4. Bake for 20 minutes.

5. While waiting, shred the rotisserie chicken.

6. Mix the broccoli florets and sour cream in a bowl.

7. Add salt and pepper and mix well.

8. Once the zucchini boats are baked, take them out and fill them with the shreds of rotisserie chicken and the broccoli florets mixture.

9. Put the cheddar cheese on top of the boats.

10. Bring the zucchini boats back into the oven and bake for 15 minutes.

11. Use the spring onion to garnish. You may even serve the zucchini boats with a bowl of keto mayonnaise.

Zucchini Nests with Pork

Prep Time: 30 minutes; **Cook Time:** 20 minutes

Serving Size: 100g; **Serves:** 4

Ingredients:

3 medium zucchinis, spiralized

4 ounces pork, chopped

¼ cup onion, chopped

¼ cup cheddar cheese, shredded

12 tablespoons sour cream

1 teaspoon garlic powder

salt and pepper

Directions:

1. Preheat oven to 350 degrees Fahrenheit.

2. Place parchment paper on a baking sheet.

3. Then, make 12 nest-like formations using the spiralized zucchinis on the baking sheet but leave a small opening in the middle of the nests.

4. Sprinkle a teaspoonful of garlic powder over the zucchinis.

5. Insert the pork, cheddar cheese and onion in the middle of the nests.

6. Bake for 20 minutes or until the zucchini's top becomes brown .

7. Put sour cream at the top of the nests before serving.

Buttered Cucumbers

Prep Time: 15-20 minutes; **Cook Time:** 5 minutes

Serving Size: 60g; **Serves:** 4

Ingredients:

2 cucumbers, peeled and sliced

3 parsley sprigs, chopped

2 ounces butter

3 tablespoons lemon juice

3 cups water

salt and pepper

Directions:

1. Put the cucumbers, water and a pinch of salt in a pot over medium heat.

2. Blanch the cucumbers for a couple of minutes.

3. Strain the excess liquid and set aside.

4. In a frying pan over low heat, put the butter and melt.

5. Add the cucumber slices and season with salt and pepper.

6. Fry the cucumbers for 3 minutes or until the edges are brown.

7. Put the fried cucumbers and lemon juice in a bowl.

8. Use the chopped parsley to garnish.

Cauliflower Mac Cheese

Prep Time: 30 minutes; **Cook Time:** 20 minutes

Serving Size: 100g; **Serves:** 4

Ingredients:

2 pounds cauliflower

8 ounces cheddar cheese, shredded

4 ounces cream cheese

1 cup heavy whipping cream

1 teaspoon turmeric

1 teaspoon mustard

½ teaspoon garlic powder

salt and pepper

Directions:

1. Put the cauliflower in a pot over medium heat. Fill the pot with water. Bring it to a boil.

2. Drain the cauliflower and set aside.

3. Place the whipping cream in a pan, heat it and wait until it simmers.

4. Add the cream cheese to the pan. Stir the mixture using a whisk.

5. Once the mixture looks smooth, put 6 ounces of cheddar cheese and set aside the remaining 2 ounces for later use. Keep on stirring until the shredded cheddar cheese melts.

6. Add salt, pepper, turmeric, mustard and garlic powder. Stir until the entire mixture becomes yellow.

7. Put the well-drained cauliflower into the pan and mix until each floret is coated with the sauce.

8. Add the remaining cheddar cheese and stir until it melts.

9. Transfer to a serving dish.

Gluten-Free Cauliflower Rice

Prep Time: 20 minutes; **Cook Time:** 7 minutes

Serving Size: 100g; **Serves:** 1-2

Ingredients:

2 cauliflower heads, finely chopped

2 tablespoons fish sauce

2 tablespoons olive oil

1 tablespoon ginger, minced

2 teaspoons garlic, minced

Directions:

1. Put the olive oil in a large pan over medium heat.

2. Toss in the garlic and ginger and sauté for a minute.

3. Add the finely chopped cauliflowers and cook over high heat for 3 minutes.

4. Put the fish sauce in the pan and cook for another 3 minutes. The cooked cauliflower will have a consistency of rice by then.

5. Serve it in a serving dish. Pair the cauliflower rice with another dish from this book.

Cauliflower Quesadillas

Prep Time: 40 minutes; **Cook Time:** 30 minutes

Serving Size: 150g; **Serves:** 4

Ingredients:

¼ cup keto mayonnaise

1½ tablespoons jalapeños in water

½ teaspoon paprika

¼ teaspoon garlic powder

1 pinch cayenne pepper

2 pounds cauliflower florets

3 eggs

¾ cup mozzarella cheese, shredded

1 cup cheddar cheese, shredded

½ teaspoon salt

Directions:

1. In a bowl, mix mayonnaise, jalapeños in water, paprika, garlic powder and cayenne pepper to make the sauce.

2. Cover the mixture and refrigerate (preferably overnight).

3. Put the cauliflower and a bit of water in a blender or food processor.

4. Pulse until it turns as sticky as rice.

5. Transfer it to another container and microwave for 10 minutes.

6. As you wait, preheat oven to 400 degrees Fahrenheit and prepare two parchment paper lined baking sheets.

7. When the cauliflower is cooked, transfer it to a towel or cheese cloth to squeeze out the excess liquid.

8. Put the cauliflower in a mixing bowl along with the mozzarella cheese, eggs and salt.

9. Stir the mixture until the cheese and eggs are well-incorporated.

10. Flatten the mixture into four circles on the baking sheets.

11. Bake for 10 minutes.

12. Flip the mixture over and bake for 6 minutes.

13. Let it cool for at least 10 minutes.

14. Coat the top of the cauliflower tortillas with the sauce.

15. Spread ¼ cup cheddar cheese to each cauliflower tortilla and then fold in half.

16. Fry each side for two minutes before flipping over.

17. Transfer to a serving dish.

Cauliflower Casserole

Prep Time: 30 minutes; **Cook Time:** 45 minutes

Serving Size: 150g; **Serves:** 2

Ingredients:

1½ cups cauliflower florets

1½ cups cheese

1 green bell pepper, diced

1 red bell pepper, diced

1 jalapeño, diced

½ white onion

1 teaspoon chili powder

1 teaspoon cumin

olive oil

Directions:

1. Preheat oven to 350 degrees Fahrenheit.

2. Cook the peppers, onion, chili powder and cumin in a skillet over medium heat until the peppers are roasted. Set aside and allow it to cool.

3. Use a blender of food processor to transform the cauliflower florets into puree. Transfer the pureed cauliflower into a microwave-safe container.

4. Microwave the cauliflower for 3 minutes.

5. Once cooked, remove the cauliflower from the microwave and add the cheese and roasted pepper mixture. Mix them well and then place them in an oiled baking sheet.

6. Bake in the preheated oven for 35 minutes.

Artichokes in Raspberry Vinaigrette

Prep Time: 25 minutes; **Cook Time:** 45-48 minutes

Serving Size: 120g; **Serves:** 4

Ingredients:

4 artichoke globes

8½ tablespoons raspberry vinaigrette

½ lemon

salt

Directions:

1. Get rid of the artichokes' rough outer leaves.

2. Cut the steam and rub the artichoke's base with the lemon.

3. Fill ¾ of a pot with water, 1 teaspoon salt and the juice from the lemon.

4. Place the pot over medium heat. Bring it to a boil.

5. Add the artichokes and cooked for 40 minutes or until the vegetables are tender.

6. Remove the artichokes from the pot and drain the water. Set aside to cool.

7. Prepare the serving dish and raspberry vinaigrette as you wait.

8. Once the artichokes are cool, remove the chokes one by one and put them on the serving dish.

9. Pour over the raspberry vinaigrette before serving.

Spinach Herb Wrap

Prep Time: 30 minutes; **Cook Time:** 10-12 minutes

Serving Size: 180g; **Serves:** 2

Ingredients:

2 cups spinach leaves

4 leaves basil, chopped

5 whole eggs

3 egg whites

1 teaspoon olive oil

1 teaspoon sesame oil

½ teaspoon salt

½ cup goat cheese, crumbled

Directions:

1. To make the wrap, put the whole eggs, egg whites, sesame oil and salt in a bowl. Mix for a minute or until it turns foamy.

2. Put half of the mixture in a preheated nonstick pan over medium heat. Cook until the entire egg mix solidifies. Set aside in a plate.

Repeat steps 1 and 2 for the remaining half of the egg mixture to form the second wrap.

3. Using the same pan, put the spinach and cook for about a minute. Set aside.

4. In a small bowl, mix the goat cheese and olive oil.

5. Get the wraps and distribute the spinach evenly.

6. Add the goat cheese and basil over the spinach.

7. Roll the wraps and chop them accordingly.

Turkey Stuffed Mushrooms

Prep Time: 45-50 minutes; **Cook Time:** 23-25 minutes

Serving Size: 150g; **Serves:** 4

Ingredients:

20 mushroom caps

1 pound turkey, thinly sliced

1 cauliflower, chopped

¼ cup goat cheese, grated

½ cup chopped chives

2 garlic cloves, minced

2 tablespoons butter, diced into 20 pieces

1 tablespoon olive oil, melted

salt and pepper

Directions:

1. Preheat oven to 400 degrees Fahrenheit.

2. Coat the mushroom caps with the melted olive oil.

3. Spread the remaining olive oil on the baking sheet.

4. Arrange the turkey slices and mushroom caps on the baking sheet.

5. Put them in the preheated oven and bake for 15 to 17 minutes.

6. As you wait, boil water in a pot over medium heat. Put the cauliflower and cook for 8 minutes.

7. Remove the pot from heat. Drain the cauliflower.

8. Place the well-drained cauliflower in a blender or food processor, along with the cheese, garlic, salt and pepper. Blend until pureed.

9. Transfer to another bowl and set aside.

10. Get the baked mushrooms and turkey.

11. Crumble the turkey and put them in a bowl.

12. Meanwhile, fill each mushroom cap with the cauliflower mix.

13. Put one dice of butter at the top of each cauliflower filled mushroom cap.

14. Sprinkle the turkey crumbles over the stuffed mushrooms.

Snacks

Kale Chips

Prep Time: 10 minutes; **Cook Time:** 12 minutes

Serving Size: 150g; **Serves:** 1

Ingredients:

1 plate of kale, washed and dried

2 tablespoons olive oil

1 tablespoon salt

Directions:

1. Preheat oven to 350 degrees Fahrenheit.

2. Put the kale and olive oil in a Ziploc bag.

3. Shake until all the kales are coated.

4. Arrange the kales in a parchment lined baking sheet.

5. Bake for 12 minutes.

6. Take it out and put them into a bowl.

7. Season with salt. Enjoy.

Cheesy Avocado Chips

Prep Time: 20 minutes; **Cook Time:** 15-17 minutes

Serving Size: 120g; **Serves:** 2

Ingredients:

1½ Hass avocados, peeled, pitted and thinly sliced

1¼ cups parmesan cheese

3 tablespoons lemon juice

pepper

Directions:

1. Preheat oven to 350 degrees Fahrenheit.

2. Put all the ingredients in a mixing bowl.

3. Mix and mash them using a fork until smooth.

4. Prepare a parchment lined baking sheet.

5. Scoop two tablespoons of the avocado and cheese mixture and form mounds in the baking sheet.

6. Using the back of a spoon, flatten the mounds to your preferred thickness.

7. Bake the avocados for 15 to 17 minutes, or until crispy.

8. Remove from oven and let it cool.

9. Serve with your preferred keto dip.

Sour Zucchini Chips

Prep Time: 30 minutes; **Cook Time:** 2-3 hours

Serving Size: 120g; **Serves:** 2

Ingredients:

2 to 3 zucchinis, thinly sliced

2 tablespoons olive oil

2 tablespoons vinegar

salt

Directions:

1. Preheat oven to 250 degrees Fahrenheit

2. Mix the vinegar and olive oil for a few seconds.

3. In a separate bowl, place the zucchini slices and pour over the vinegar and oil mixture.

4. Sprinkle salt over the zucchini slices. Make sure each slice is coated with the vinegar and oil mix, and seasoned with salt.

5. Arrange the zucchini slices in a parchment lined baking sheet.

6. Put the baking sheet in the preheated oven for 2 to 3 hours, depending on your desired crispness and thinness of your zucchini slices.

7. Take them out of the oven and allow them to cool for 5 minutes.

8. Keep them in Ziploc bags or any similar airtight container if you are not going to consume them right away.

Cucumber Boats

Prep Time: 7-10 minutes

Serving Size: 80g; **Serves:** 1

Ingredients:

½ cucumber, peeled, halved and seeded

cream cheese (or any of your preferred fillings)

Directions:

1. Scoop cream cheese and stuff it in one cucumber half.

2. Fill it as much as you want and then cover it with the other cucumber half. You may replace the cream cheese filling with any of your preferred filling.

Cucumber and Berry Caterpillars

Prep Time: 15 minutes

Serving Size: 50g; **Serves:** 8

Ingredients:

4 cucumbers, peeled

1 cup of mixed berries (preferably raspberries, blackberries and strawberries), sliced

Directions:

1. Slice the cucumbers into half, crosswise.

2. Make cuts on the cucumbers that will serve as slots for the berry slices.

3. Insert 1 or 2 berry slices in one cut in the cucumbers.

4. Serve with your preferred keto condiment.

Berry Popsicles

Prep Time: 1 hour; **Cook Time:** 10 minutes

Serving Size: 100g; **Serves:** 6

Ingredients:

1 cup blueberries

1 cup raspberries

1 cup water

1½ cups coconut cream

1½ teaspoons Liquid Stevia

½ teaspoon vanilla extract

Directions:

1. Put the blueberries, ½ teaspoon Liquid Stevia and ½ cup water in a saucepan. Boil the mixture using medium heat for five minutes. Set aside to cool.

   In another saucepan, repeat the steps for the raspberries.

2. Get the blueberry mixture and use a blender to make it into blue puree. Do the same with the raspberry mixture to have a red puree.

3. Refrigerate the purees in their respective containers.

4. As you wait, mix the vanilla extract, ½ teaspoon Liquid Stevia and 1½ cups of coconut cream in a bowl.

5. Put the coconut cream mixture in the refrigerator and get the raspberry mixture out.

6. Put three tablespoons of the raspberry mixture on each of your popsicle molds.

7. Chill it for an hour or until the puree hardens.

8. Bring it out again and add three tablespoons of the coconut cream mixture to each mold.

9. Put in the freezer for 30 minutes.

10. After that, get them out and add stick to each of the popsicles.

11. Chill for another 30 minutes before bringing them out.

12. Add three tablespoons of the blueberry puree to each mold.

13. Chill for at least an hour before consumption.

Berry Bombs

Prep Time: 35 minutes; **Cook Time:** 5 minutes

Serving Size: 120g; **Serves:** 2

Ingredients:

½ cup blackberries (may be replaced with strawberries or raspberries)

1 cup butter

1 cup olive oil

1 tablespoon lemon juice

½ teaspoon Liquid Stevia

¼ teaspoon vanilla powder

Directions:

1. Put the butter, olive oil and berries in a pot over medium heat. Cook for 5 minutes. Stir well.

2. Remove from heat and allow the berries to cool.

3. As you wait, prepare your blender or food processor.

4. Put the remaining ingredients inside the blender or food processor.

5. Add the berries when they are cool enough to touch.

6. Blend the mixture until pureed.

7. Put the berry mixture in a parchment lined baking pan.

8. Place it in the fridge for at least an hour.

9. Cut the berry mix into your preferred shape before serving.

Tasty Cheddar Cheese Mug Cake

Prep Time: 15 minutes; **Cook Time:** 70 seconds

Serving Size: 100g; **Serves:** 1

Ingredients:

1 egg

3 tablespoons almond flour

2 tablespoons butter

2 ½ tablespoons white cheddar cheese, shredded

1 tablespoon green chili

½ teaspoon baking powder

¼ teaspoon cayenne pepper

salt and pepper

Directions:

1. Put all the ingredients (except for the pepper and ½ tablespoon of cheddar cheese) in a mug and mix.

2. Put in the microwave for 70 seconds.

3. Slightly slam the mug against the serving dish.

4. Place the remaining cheddar cheese at the top of the mug cake and sprinkle a bit of pepper.

Spicy Nachos

Prep Time: 30 minutes; **Cook Time:** 13-15 minutes

Serving Size: 150g; **Serves:** 3-4

Ingredients:

1 pound small peppers, halved and seeded

1 pound ground beef

5 green olives, chopped

1½ cups cheddar cheese, shredded

1 tablespoon chili powder

1 teaspoon garlic powder

1 teaspoon paprika

1 teaspoon ground cumin

½ teaspoon oregano

1 pinch red pepper flakes

salt and pepper

Directions:

1. Mix the chili powder, garlic powder, paprika, ground cumin, oregano and red pepper flakes in a small bowl.

2. Season the mixture with salt and pepper.

3. Put the ground beef in a skillet over medium heat. Cook for 8 to 10 minutes.

4. Put the spice mixture in the skillet and stir well.

5. Preheat oven to 400 degrees Fahrenheit.

6. Transfer the cooked ground beef in a parchment lined baking sheet.

7. Place the pepper halves in the baking sheet and sprinkle them with the shredded cheese and ground beef mixture.

8. Put in the preheated oven and bake until the cheese completely melts.

9. Take the pan out of the oven. Transfer the baked pepper nachos in a serving dish. Garnish them with the chopped green olives before serving.

Cheesy Cauliflower Sandwiches

Prep Time: 30 minutes; **Cook Time:** 25-28 minutes

Serving Size: 150g; **Serves:** 2

Ingredients:

2 cups cauliflower florets

½ cup parmesan cheese, shredded

2 cheddar cheese slices

1 large egg

salt

Directions:

1. Put the cauliflower florets in a blender or food processor. Blend until it has the consistency of rice.

2. Transfer it to a microwave-safe container and microwave for a couple of minutes.

3. Stir the cauliflower and put it back in the microwave. Microwave the cauliflowers for a further 3 minutes.

4. Remove the cauliflowers, stir and microwave again for a further 5 minutes. Transfer it to a bowl and set aside to cool.

5. Preheat oven to 450 degrees Fahrenheit.

6. Mix the parmesan cheese and egg. Season the mixture with salt.

7. Add the cauliflowers and mix well until it turns paste-like.

8. Divide the mixture into four. Place them into a parchment lined baking sheet. Flatten and form them into four squares.

9. Bake for 15 to 18 minutes. The cauliflower mixture will serve as the bread or crust for your sandwich.

10. Insert the cheddar cheese slice between two baked cauliflower crusts.

11. You can eat them like that or you may opt to bake the sandwiches first in a toaster oven.

Pork-Wrapped Jalapeño Bites

Prep Time: 30 minutes; **Cook Time:** 20 minutes

Serving Size: 50g; **Serves:** 8

Ingredients:

14 ounces pork, cut into 16 strips

16 jalapeños

4 ounces cream cheese

¼ cup cheddar cheese, shredded

1 teaspoon paprika

1 teaspoon salt

Directions:

1. Preheat oven to 350 degrees Fahrenheit.

2. Wear gloves and then cut each jalapeño length-wise.

3. Cut the stem and scoop out the seeds and membrane in each jalapeño half.

4. To make the filling, mix the cheeses in one bowl.

5. Stuff the jalapeño halves with the cheese mixture.

6. Put together two jalapeño halves and wrap a pork strip around them. Do this for the rest of the jalapeños.

7. Put all of them in a foil lined baking sheet and bake for 20 minutes.

8. Arrange the baked jalapeños in a serving dish and sprinkle paprika and salt over them before serving.

Tasty Queso Fresco Cubes

Prep Time: 15 minutes; **Cook Time:** 16-18 minutes

Serving Size: 100g; **Serves:** 4

Ingredients:

1 pound queso fresco, cubed

½ tablespoon olive oil

1 tablespoon coconut oil

Directions:

1. Put the olive oil and coconut oil in a pan over high heat.

2. Once the oils smoke, add the cubes of queso fresco.

3. Cook each side until browned before flipping over to another side.

4. Use paper towel to remove the extra oils.

Flavored Cheese Chips

Prep Time: 15 minutes; Cook Time: 10 minutes

Serving Size: 100g; Serves: 2

Ingredients:

1½ ounces cheddar cheese, shredded

3 tablespoons ground flaxseed

your preferred seasonings

Directions:

1. Preheat oven to 425 degrees Fahrenheit.

2. Get 2 tablespoons of cheddar cheese and form them into mounds on a non-stick pan.

3. Sprinkle the ground flaxseed over the cheese mounds.

4. Sprinkle or spread over your favorite seasonings.

5. Put the pan in the preheated oven and bake for 10 minutes.

6. Allow the cheese chips to cool. Refer to the Condiments section to make the dip for your cheese chips.

Chapter 6: Post- Cleanse

Reaching the last day of your cleansing period without eating the foods that you should avoid is a feat in itself. However, it does not mean that you can let your guard down and entertain the prospect of eating the foods you avoided and ditching the keto meals you ate in the last two weeks. Just like transitioning to keto cleansing meals, returning to regular diet can also turn out to be difficult.

What to Expect

The effects of dieting differ from one person to another. Some reported feeling light and happy while some felt grumpy and weak after the cleansing period. One thing is for certain though: you are bound to feel hungry especially on the last two to three days. Eating snacks every three hours help tone down the hunger during the cleansing period. However, the post-cleansing period is another story.

Your hunger may trigger your binge eating tendency after the cleansing period. If you give in, you will end up wasting your efforts in the last 15 days. The best way to deal with this is proper preparation.

What to Do After the Cleansing Period

Start your transition by drinking lemon-infused water in the morning. To make your own infused water, simply fill your tumbler with water and a few slices of lemon. Put it in the fridge for at least 30 minutes before drinking. You may also mix and match different fruits, vegetables, spices and herbs.

Stick to keto meals as well to have it ingrained in your system. Once ingrained, you can treat yourself with non-keto but still nutritious foods every now and then. Going back to keto meals will no longer be as hard as when you first started out.

It also pays to consume probiotics like goat milk and yogurt to further strengthen your gut. It helps to eat sauerkraut, pickles, soup and steamed vegetables as well. Avoid cold beverages for the meantime and make sure you still eat every three hours, much like during your cleansing period.

Relaxation techniques like deep breathing, mindfulness, meditation and yoga can also keep distractive thoughts at bay during and after the 15 days of cleansing. Aside from that, they also help you eliminate toxic and pessimistic thoughts. After all, both the body and soul need nourishment and cleansing.

Conclusion

Thank you again for downloading this book!

I hope this book was able to help you carry out a 15-day ketogenic dieting program with delicious and nourishing meals. Hopefully, the recipes and advice in this book made the cleansing period an enjoyable and enlightening experience. You can now go back to a regular diet but with safer and more nutritious meals instead of your unhealthy choices in the past. Take the cleansing period as the start of your journey to better wellness.

The next step is to sustain all the healthy eating habits you developed while on the cleansing period. Refer to this book when you cleanse again after four months at the very least.

Thank you and good luck!